SPIRITUAL INSIGHTS *into* Nutrition and Chronic Diseases

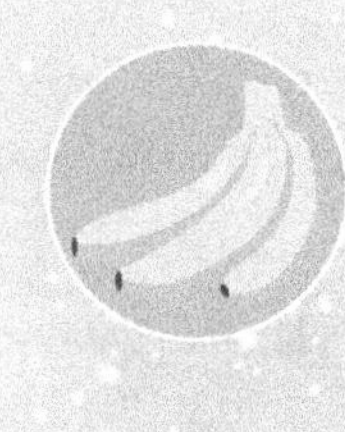

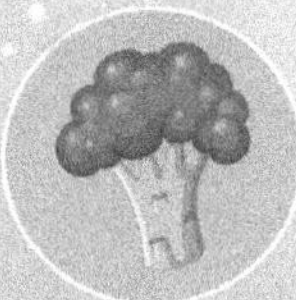

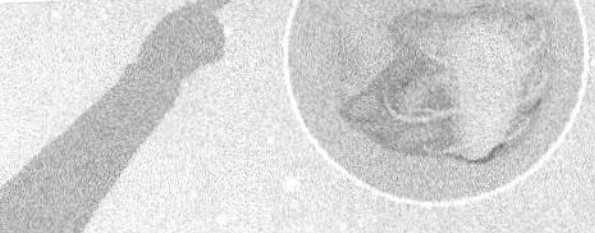

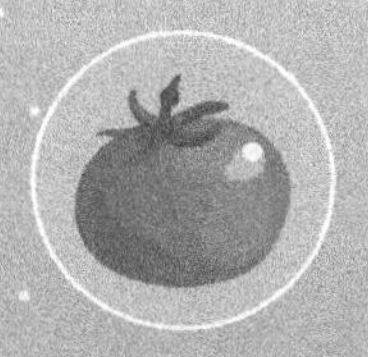

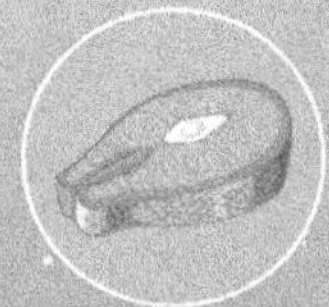

RACHEL NOAMESHIE

Spiritual Insights *into* "Nutrition and Chronic Diseases"
First Edition

ISBN: 979-8-218-42527-2

Printed in the United States of America

SPIRITUAL INSIGHTS

into

"Nutrition and Chronic Diseases"

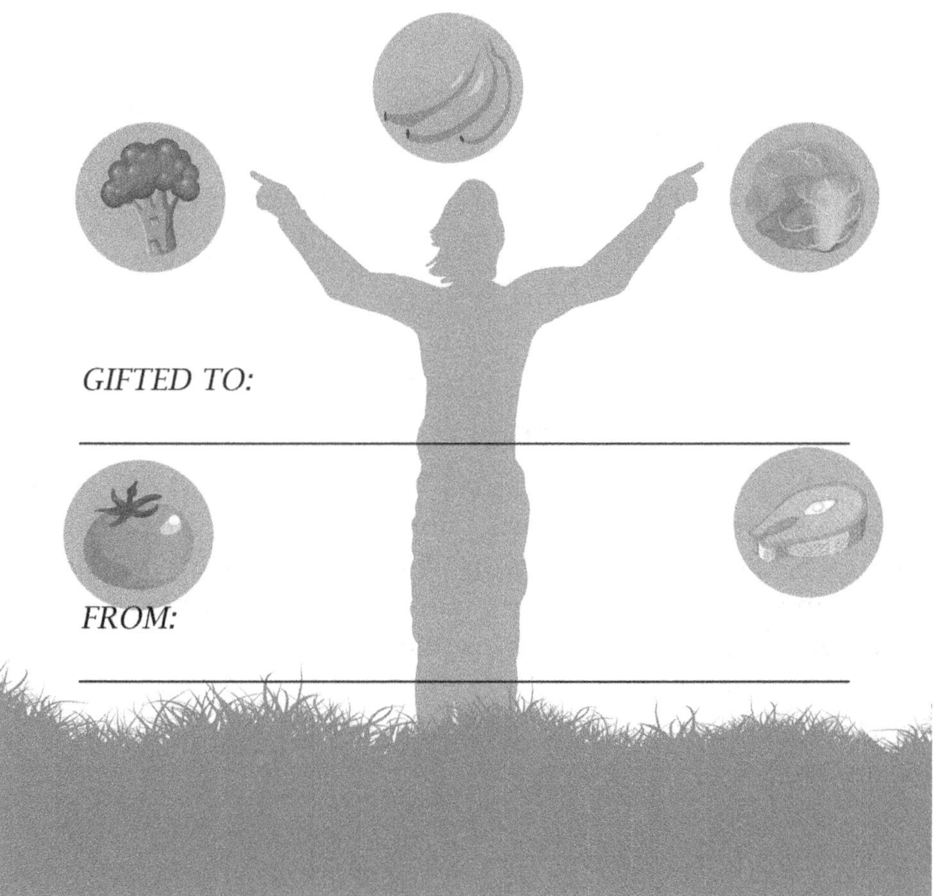

GIFTED TO:

FROM:

DEDICATION

This book is dedicated to every Bible Believer battling any form of metabolic illness or struggling with an unhealthy lifestyle.

A Special Thank You to the following individuals:

Pastor Favour and Prophet Corry Robinson, whose insights helped shake me out of my unproductive thoughts and actions.

The Taylors; especially Mrs. Nicole Taylor, who supported my soul-healing journey.

Pastor Kevin LA Ewing, whose teachings deepened my understanding of the spiritual realm as per the scriptures.

Mrs. Marlene Baugh, whose vast network seems to know no bounds.

My sisters Lauren and Muriel Noameshie, for their continuous check-ins and encouragement.

I am immensely grateful to my **Heavenly Father** for **His** numerous blessings, **His** grace, and **His** patience, which even extends to **His** sense of humor. I am deeply thankful for the transformative and exhilarating journey of knowing my **Lord** and **Savior Jesus Christ**, and for all the people **He** placed in my life to make this book a reality.

God bless each one of you for your contributions.

Thank You!

CONTENTS

INTRODUCTION

I just heard a woman of God say that the first sin was committed with food. Indeed! Satan orchestrated man's fall by way of a fruit ... by way of food.

I then understood why the Lord put this book in my heart. Food overall plays a heavy spiritual role in terms of a weapon used by the enemy. Unfortunately, many believers see food and our interaction with food to be absolutely harmless. Food from my perspective is looked at by many God-loving bible believers to be innocent. That is a dangerous mistake.

1 Corinthians 10:23 NKJV - "All things are lawful [a]for me, but not all things are helpful; all things are lawful for me, but not all things [b]edify."

1 Corinthians 10:23 AMP - "All things are lawful [that is, morally legitimate, permissible], but not all things are beneficial or advantageous. All things are lawful, but not all things are constructive [to character] and edifying [to spiritual life].

I have always struggled with the believer's mentality of *"freedom"* while indulging in self-destructive behaviors. I always wonder about the rationale behind living a blatantly unhealthy lifestyle, and then going to God to pray for healing: As His children, we may pray; *"Lord I am going to trash my body and treat this temple anyhow, but please heal me, please heal this body while I am trashing it."* That's the unhealthy *mantra* some of His children practice.

Brothers and sisters, IT DOESN'T WORK THAT WAY.

I am not saying that God doesn't help or heal (His mercy is beyond comprehension), but God doesn't encourage self-destructive behaviors: that is against His very loving nature. That is against His very will that we prosper (3 John 1:2.) That is against His very good thoughts towards us (Jeremiah 29:11.) But most importantly, that is against His order. 1 Corinthians 14: 33, 40.

Understand that I am not talking about illnesses that do not have a preventable basis per scientific or medical standards. For example, obesity and smoking are well-known risk factors for cancer, however, not everyone who deals with cancer is obese or has ever smoked. These types of situations typically call on investigating deeper spiritual root causes or sometimes occupational exposures (which I consider setups; your profession should not set you up for death.) I am not talking about contributing causes that are a bit less evident to prevent, such as heart or kidney defects at birth (which doesn't rule out the healing ministry of Jesus Christ and even having to investigate and alienate the cause.) Regardless, God heals and is a Healer.

If you assess that your state of health is the result of a curse, the Scriptures say that a curse without a cause will not take effect (Proverbs 26:2); therefore, if there is a curse taking effect in your life, what is the cause? In this instance, you should be investigating, confronting, and alienating any root cause to the curses or "non-modifiable factors" (again, non-modifiable per medical, human standards, not God's.) I am talking about evil foundations, evil altars, evil covenants.... (2 Corinthians 10:4.) The weapons of our warfare are not carnal. Contending for your health is a form of warfare in these days and ages. As a matter of fact, in biblical times, King Hezekiah contended for his healing and got 15 years added to his life (2 Kings 20:5-6.) Anything that takes place in the physical has already taken place in the spiritual. We have been given the authority to address what is against us (Luke 10:19); as the fight is not carnal.

This is why the enemy has come up with a way to insert diseases into your life while making you think that it is natural, acceptable, or worse; normal. When you are sick or not well in your body, a bulk of your prayer life would be directed towards that specific deficit when there are so many other things to address and intercede for. Sickness is nothing more than a direct assault from the enemy to move us away from our purpose and destiny. The Lord has need of you. (Mark 11:3-paraphrased). The sickness often is a powerful distraction, and it often turns you into a selfish believer. Your health may even impede your prayer life and the mission you are supposed to accomplish on this earth. An easy way for the enemy to destroy the ones that he cannot easily seduce with a worldly life is through a (not so evident) unhealthy lifestyle. Moreover, it is very easy for him to seduce any believer who lacks discernment through food. Many aspects of that lifestyle may have been passed on from generation to generation, so it is considered *"normal."*

This book is about preventative lifestyle illnesses. The ones most of us can avoid with applied knowledge; especially when we decide not to subscribe to the narrative of *"obesity is common now, there is a medication for that,"* or *"hypertension is not unusual, or it runs in my family, there is a medication for that,"* or *"I too have the sugar aka type II diabetes, to be exact."*

I once heard someone say: knowledge is not power. It is the application of knowledge which is power. As far as I am concerned, that individual was right on the money.

3 John 1:2 NLT - "Dear friend, I hope all is well with you and you are as healthy in body as you are strong in spirit.". The NKJV version reads: **"Beloved, I pray that you**

may prosper in all things and be in health just as your soul prospers."

When I decided to take my health seriously (I was in my early to mid-30s); this scripture was a pillar for me. Why? Stress or Emotional eating. I was a stress / emotional eater. I ate for comfort when upset, and I ate to celebrate. The interesting thing is that when you eat in reaction to an emotional state you typically eat things that are not necessarily good for you. Moreover, you overeat the not-so-beneficial food especially if the eating action is carried out in the pursuit of some type of comfort. *"I pray that you may prosper and be in good health ...."*

Although I am a nurse practitioner by training, I will insist that some of the information here will not be scientifically evidence-based because it is coming from a place of conviction and scriptures. Scriptures are way ahead of science which eventually catches up with findings (or whenever it is deemed necessary for disclosure.) At that point, one who is led to understand the scriptures with the help of the **Holy Spirit** can't help but exclaim *"This is why such and such is in the Bible"* or *"This has been in the Bible for ages! How is that a discovery?"* And even *"Umm that is what this scripture meant."*

I have this personal conviction that all answers are in the Bible. **PERIOD.**

When it comes to your diet (and by diet, I mean eating habits.) I hope that this book helps you approach self-sabotaging behaviors from a spiritual perspective, and how it translates naturally. If you find yourself turning in a circle and being unable to defeat the harmful behaviors you have identified and know you need to rid of, you very likely need to take it to the spiritual level. Example *"Oh, I must have at least one coke every day."* You do know that Coke is one of the best toilet bowl cleaners, right? Try it.

2 Corinthians 10:4-6 KJV – "For the weapons of our warfare are not carnal, but mighty through God to the pulling down of strongholds. Casting down imaginations, and every high thing that exalted itself against the knowledge of God and bringing into captivity every thought to the obedience of Christ. And having in a readiness to revenge all disobedience, when your obedience is fulfilled."

Note: We have some powerful weapons through God, one being "casting down imagination and every high thing that promotes itself against the knowledge of God." Knowledge in Hebrew *"dah'ath"* means perception, discernment, understanding wisdom. The NLT version sums it up: "We use God's mighty weapons, not worldly weapons to knock down the strongholds of human reasoning and to destroy false arguments."

- In Greek, knowledge is *"gnosis"* it signifies intelligence and understanding. It denotes a certain level of discernment. When you truly know somebody, you recognize them, you identify them in the crowd of a multitude! So the understanding of God's word, will, heart, and way of operation can only come from a true intimate relationship with God. From there you can isolate imaginations and every high thing that is not God. This exemplifies the knowledge of God.

1

What Are Lifestyle Illnesses?

Simply put, Lifestyle Illnesses are illnesses or conditions often caused by the choices influenced by our lifestyles. Those include hypertension, diabetes, high cholesterol, and as far as I am concerned any complication that follows. In medicine, these conditions are also put in the category of preventable illnesses.

I believe preventative illnesses to be a result of a lifestyle coming from our imagination and high things that are not from God.

We know that some complications from uncontrolled hypertension include kidney diseases (to the point of end-stage renal failure, and therefore Dialysis), heart failure, and some forms of dementia.

Exodus 15:26 NIV - "If you listen carefully to the Lord your God and do what is right in his eyes if you pay attention to his commands and keep all his decrees, I will not bring on

you any of the diseases I brought on the Egyptians, for I am the Lord, who heals you."

Deuteronomy 7:15 KJV - "And the Lord will take away from thee all sickness, and will put none of the evil diseases of Egypt, which though knowest, upon thee; but will lay them upon all of them that hate thee."

Deuteronomy 34:7 NASB 1995 – "Although Moses was one hundred and twenty years old when he died, his eye was not dim, nor his vigor abated."

Matthew 8:17 NASB 1995 – "This was to fulfill what was spoken through Isaiah the prophet: "He Himself took our infirmities and carried away our diseases."

An Example Of Hypertension:

I recently had a conversation with a young man in his 30s who battled hypertension. His statement was as follows: *"Everybody has hypertension in my family, my parents have heart problems…etc."* I asked him: *"Do you want to have hypertension?"* To which he replied, *"Of course not."* I replied, *"Then, why are you subscribing to the narrative, be the proof that hypertension doesn't have to run in your family."*

Although he was an athletic and mindful eater, we discussed stress management, eating habits, sleeping habits, weight, and exercise, and I shared some scriptures with him in terms of God takes no pleasure in His children being sick. In a couple of months, the high blood pressure he had dealt with since his teenage years was nearly normalized. One thing I mentioned to him was the importance of listening to our bodies. There are general guidelines and rules out there, however, we each are different. I explained to him that with his sleeping habits, his response to stress, and even his eating choices, he is to note how his body reacts, and how he feels. That is how he establishes what works for him. And by listening to your body, I mean your being, you are not only paying attention to how it reacts, but truly you are listening to the Inward Witness of the **Holy Spirit.** This as a lifestyle can only be for your benefit.

APPLICATION:

As a Bible believer, these are general questions you should ask yourself when it comes to your lifestyle.

- How does my body react (how do I feel) when I eat certain foods?

- Do I notice some symptoms? If so, when do I notice my symptoms are worse?

- What drives me to indulge in harmful habits? WHY? HOW?

- Do I have self-control?

- What narrative do I tell myself about the illnesses in question? Do I buy into those narratives?

- Do I move enough?

- Do I sleep well?

- Do I sleep enough?

- How does my circle affect my choices? Do I need to make some changes in this area (circle)?

- Have I ever gone to **God** with this struggle? What did **He** say? Did I apply **His** instructions?

2

Stress Or Emotional Eating (Overindulgence/Gluttony)

Typically, stress eating manifests in two ways, under-eating or over/binge eating. According to the **National Institute of Health**, *"Binge-eating disorder is a condition where people lose control over their eating and have reoccurring episodes of eating unusually large amounts of food. Unlike bulimia nervosa, periods of binge eating are not followed by purging, excessive exercise, or fasting. As a result, people with binge-eating disorders often are overweight or obese.*[1]*"*

I am addressing bingeing and overeating because of the correlation with obesity or excessive weight which is gaining ground.

Eve had access to all the food in the Garden of Eden. Unfortunately, she didn't deem it necessary to resist the temptation when the fruit of the forbidden tree was suggested to

---

1 https://www.nimh.nih.gov/health/topics/eating-disorders.

her, greed kicked in, especially at the tantalizing idea of being like God.

There is a certain level of greed behind stress eating: *"I am going to eat this much to feel good, or I am going to keep eating to keep experiencing the pleasure it is giving me."*

Proverbs 25:16 KJV – "Hast thou found honey? eat so much as is sufficient for thee, lest thou be filled therewith and vomit it."

Proverbs 25:16 NLT – "Do you like honey? Do not eat it too much or it will make you sick!" This scripture alone is enough and doesn't require me to expand on this chapter (ha-ha) nevertheless, let me elaborate.

Philippians 4:6-7 KJV – "**Be careful for nothing**; but in every thing by prayer and supplication with thanksgiving let your requests be made known unto God. And the peace of God, which passeth all understanding, shall keep your hearts and minds through Christ Jesus."

Philippians 4:6-7 ESV – "**do not be anxious about anything**, but in everything by prayer and supplication with thanksgiving let your requests be made known to God. And the peace of God which surpasses all understanding, will guard your hearts and your minds in Christ Jesus."

The scriptures inform us to make our requests known unto God with prayer and supplication, it further states that the PEACE of God which SURPASSES ALL UNDERSTANDING will keep your heart and minds through Christ. That peace is what prevents you from getting into that emotional state where you make wrong decisions including with food. That peace keeps you in Christ which means you are protected and shielded. Not only that; it says in verse 5 to let your moderation be known unto all men because the Lord is at hand. Keyword: *"Moderation."* Now let us examine it in the context of eating.

The word *moderation* in the original Greek is "*epieikēs*" which means seemly, suitable, equitable, fair, middle, and gentle. The way I understand moderation from those words is an *"appropriate, fit."*

Proverbs 25:16 KJV – "Hast thou found honey? Eat so much as is sufficient for thee, lest thou be filled therewith and vomit it." NLT – "Do you like honey? Do not eat it too much or it will make you sick!"

When we deal with nausea and vomiting after ingesting something, we would say that whatever we ingested *"isn't sitting right"* or *"not agreeing with my body/stomach."* Indeed, in the context of Proverbs 25:16, you vomit the surplus or the amount that your body wouldn't take. But why wouldn't your body take it? Because it wasn't designed that way. Why wasn't it designed that way; beyond the obvious fact that when you fill a bottle up the excess runs over and out of the bottle? Because it doesn't honor God! As in:

1 Corinthians 6:20 NLT – "For God bought you with a high price. So you must honor God with your body. How do I know it doesn't honor God? It is said in Proverbs 23:2 KJV – "And put a knife to your throat if thou be a man given to appetite." "Given appetite" – no control of appetite: that is how much being an *"overindulgent/glutton"* disqualifies you.

The Hebrew, the word for "appetite" is *nep̄eš* which means soul, self, life, creature, person appetite, mind, living being, desire, emotion, and passion.

My God: When you are stressed or overeating, you are making food an idol. You are putting creation in lieu of God. You are letting that desire which must first be a thought let itself exalt above the very knowledge of God and what He said.

You are overindulging in creation while disobeying **His** instructions for moderation. The pleasure it provides you, your soul, your being is more important than the peace you are supposed to get from applying **Philippians 4:7**. That very peace that prevents you from practicing any form of idolatry (self, soul, creature…) as it guards your heart and emotions through **Christ.** Mind you, the peace obtained from overindulgence/gluttony is very fleeting and is often followed by an uneasy feeling (even if you deny it). Your spirit lets you know that something isn't right with that behavior (until you fully silence your spirit if you are stubborn enough): We are masters at justifying our misbehaviors and silencing the **Holy Spirit** witnessing to us inwardly.

I should not even call it misbehavior; or neither should I call it sin. It is iniquity. That stubbornness to keep going against the word is iniquity (**1 Samuel 15:23**). When you continue to go back and repeat the sin; it is iniquity. Note that iniquity goes throughout generations, but I will cover that in the *Epigenetics*[2] Chapter.

Every time you are stress eating you are worshipping another god. Food in its natural state is creation. Food when we create/perform recipes or however we make things edible is man-made, just like any wooden representation of something or any creation such as wind, fire, or sun.

According to the *Mayo Clinic,* your strongest cravings sometimes occur when you are at your lowest emotionally. Yet, we have **Philippians 4:7**. I am not saying that we never have lows, the Prophet Elijah was so depressed he wanted to die, but you know how that story ends. Do not let your lows rule your life and keep

---

[2] Epigenetics is the study of how cells control gene activity without changing the DNA sequence."Epi-"means on or above in Greek,and "epigenetic" describes factors beyond the genetic code. Epigenetic changes are modifications to DNA that regulate whether genes are turned on or off.

you in iniquity. There are several obvious ways for this to happen (being in iniquity that is), but oftentimes, we do not realize that our eating behavior is also one of the ways of being in iniquity. A very subtle yet powerful way.

PS: I didn't say food is evil; it's the love of food that is evil.

How many times does **God** talk about feasting in the Bible? However, it should be noted, that it's the **RIGHT FOODS IN MODERATION.**

APPLICATION:

- Confront the thought and idea when it occurs. Cast it down.

- Remind yourself of why stress eating is a harmful response to stress on different levels (spiritually, emotionally, and then physically).

- You may need deliverance and counseling.

- Find healthy stress-relieving activities (exercise, music, dance, social company, or even getting some rest if you are sleep-deprived). Did you know that the more tired and exhausted the more likely to eat unhealthily and overindulge?

- When do you notice your lows occur? Are there any events or seasons associated with it? If so, have you addressed those?

- Counseling may help you identify the abnormal ways you may be dealing with a situation with the wrong perspective. However, you want to go to the root. By prayer and fasting.

- FORGIVE, FORGIVE, FORGIVE. You may need to forgive by Faith until it becomes tangible but forgive; Choose to forgive. Unforgiveness is caging your mind, spirit, and soul. It helps fuel all kinds of issues, including the issues of the heart.

- God knew what He was doing when He was teaching us to forgive.

Matthew 6:14-15 NLT – "If you forgive those who sin against you, your heavenly Father will forgive you, but if you refuse to forgive others, your Father will not forgive your sins."

Can you imagine the guilt and torment level your spirit carries from not forgiving others? Our Father doesn't contradict Himself; His word is bond and He said He cannot forgive you unless you do so of others. Our spirit is carrying that weight which manifests also in the natural as depression (interestingly depression feels like being weighted, or bogged down). You carry stress when you have not forgiven.

- A life of sincere repentance (which also entails turning from the wrong ways); is golden. Ask King David (well he is gone, but you can read about him in the scriptures and find out).

3

Processed Food

What sort of imagination gave birth to processed food? Was it Godly or was it a high imagination? According to the ***Department of Agriculture***[3], processed food is any raw agricultural commodities that have been washed, cleaned, milled, cut, chopped, heated, pasteurized, blanched, cooked, canned, frozen, dried, dehydrated, mixed or packaged —in other words, anything done to the foods that alter their natural state. This may include adding preservatives, flavors, nutrients, and other food additives, or substances approved for use in food products, such as salt, sugars, and fats. ***The Institute of Food Technologists***[4] includes additional processing terms like "storing, filtering, fermenting, extracting, concentrating, microwaving, and packaging."

---

[3] https://www.hsph.harvard.edu/nutritionsource/processed-foods/#:~:text=The%20U.S.%20Department%20of%20Agriculture,%2C%20drying%2C%20dehydrating%2C%20mixing%2C

[4] https://www.hsph.harvard.edu/nutritionsource/processed-foods/#:~:text=The%20U.S.%20Department%20of%20Agriculture,%2C%20drying%2C%20dehydrating%2C%20mixing%2C

According to these standards, virtually all foods sold in the supermarket would be classified as *"processed"* to some degree. Because food begins to deteriorate and loses nutrients as soon as it is harvested, even the apple in the produce aisle undergoes four or more processing steps before being sold to the consumer. That's why in practice, it's helpful to differentiate between the various degrees of food processing.

Depending on where we live and what we have access to (farmer's market in the US vs organic food in Africa), we will have to make do and minimize our exposure to processed food to the best of our abilities especially when it comes to food additives, and this is why:

Many of today's processed foods have elements and additives that get you *"hooked"* to whatever the food is. So you find yourself always wanting that. After all, the goal of those additives (MSG, Refined Flour, Refined Sugar, Gluten, etc.…) is to not only make you crave that food but also make you hungrier altogether by how it influences your brain response (the brain sends the craving signals; you want to eat that food although you are not hungry or shouldn't be eating it).

According to the ***World Health Organization,*** food additives are substances not normally consumed as food by themselves and not normally used as typical ingredients in food.

Think about folks who say they do not drink water, but they drink soda. What did mankind drink before the creation of soda? Do you mean that you would have died of thirst? Anyways, you constantly go to those processed foods, not occasionally, nor in moderation. In other words, food additives initiate many into idolatry as they cannot control those cravings and make those foods their idols by overindulging. How many practice 2 Cor. 10:5 by casting down those vain imaginations (passion) as we mentioned in the introduction?

Colossians 3:5 NLT – "So put to death the sinful, earthly things **lurking within you.** Have nothing to do with sexual immorality, impurity, lust, and evil desires. Don't be greedy, for a greedy person is an idolater and worshipping the things of this world."

KJV version says – "Mortify, therefore, your members which are upon the earth; fornication, uncleanness, **inordinate affection**, evil concupiscence, and covetousness, which is idolatry."

One of the definitions of greed per the **Merriam-Webster Dictionary** is *"having a strong desire for food or drink (ha!)"*

Let me reiterate: The introduction of someways of processed foods is not innocent from a spiritual perspective. Many are not aware of the agenda and do not feel the initiative to dominate or conquer those cravings (some may need deliverance altogether). As mentioned earlier, the Bible says, "a curse causeless shall not take effect."-paraphrased. Yet, you find yourself practicing idolatry of foods, bringing curses on yourself, and then wonder why you are dealing with certain health conditions. From the natural perspective, food additives are linked to many conditions that I will lightly explain in the next chapter as this subject is a whole dictionary-sized book on its own.

APPLICATION:

- The more natural and closer to the original state, the better the food is for you (I am not telling you to eat only raw food unless you feel led to.)

- The less processed food in your diet the better for you (haven't you been hearing this?) Don't overindulge in them, minimize them, and eliminate them if circumstances allow.

4

Inflammation is a Curse: Are you "Cursing" Yourself?

Deuteronomy 28:22 KJV – "The Lord shall smite thee with a consumption, **and** with a fever, **and** with an inflammation, **and** with an extreme burning, **and** with the sword, **and** with blasting **and** with mildew, **and** they shall pursue thee until thou perish."

- Consumption: The Hebrew word *Sahepet* means wasting disease, wasting disease of the lungs.
- Fever: Hebrew word *qadahat:* burning *ague* (fever with shiver).
- Inflammation: Hebrew word *Dalleqet:* burning fever.
- Extreme burning: Hebrew word *Harhur*: extreme heat, inflammation, violent heat, fever.

I first wondered why fever is used in so many different manners. Then I understood, that there are different degrees of fever involved. Consumption is a wasting disease, that **could range** from degenerative muscle conditions **to** COPD[5], and such. It doesn't necessarily involve a high temperature. However, the curse **IS** consumption **and** fever (not or fever), **and** inflammation (not or inflammation), **and** extreme burning (not or extreme burning).

So, while one may be dealing with consumption, there is inflammation, fever, and extreme burning happening at least from a spiritual perspective. It is just a matter of manifesting. Is it not interesting that individuals with Rheumatoid Arthritis (RA) sometimes experience fever (fever as we know it)?

How does one develop psoriatic arthritis from psoriasis which affects the skin and nails? I have taken care of patients with "uncontrolled" psoriatic arthritis. These patients experience, very painful swelling and locking of the joints in addition to skin anomalies.

Science defines inflammation as *"the body's immune system's response to an irritant."* It's the body reacting to something interfering with its well-being, well-functioning, etc… That is the physical manifestation of fever and the scientific definition. When you are dealing with inflammation, in the spiritual world, your being is burning by fever because of a "foreign agent." The issue with this is that the burning is not selective, and this can result in your demise.

However with inflammatory conditions, although you may not be dealing with a distinctive fever, your body is still dealing with something it considers doesn't belong, the core temperature is very subtly raised and still has negative outcomes in the long term. Let's think about arthritis, psoriasis, and so on. To control

---

[5] Definition: Chronic Obstructive Pulumonary Diseases.

these, one will often find themselves on pharmacologic regimens (often immunosuppressors or weakeners of the immune system) and usually with side effects.

When you look closely at Deut. 28:22 KJV version, inflammation is essentially a curse with different levels and types of inflammations.

In one of my YouTube videos, I expound on the types of foods to minimize or avoid when you deal with inflammation. In summary:

Processed Foods: According to the *University of Chicago Medicin*e,[6] processed foods can interfere with the behavior of our gut bacteria yet our gut is heavily involved in our immune system. Processed foods are the worst at creating the mechanism leading to inflammation by making our guts more permeable, which allows bacteria and other inflammatory particles into our bloodstream more easily.

Refined Processed Sugars: Sugars and other inflammatory foods cause our *"bad"* cholesterol (LDL) to rise, which leads to more C-reactive protein (CRP). CRP is a protein, its expression increases with inflammatory conditions such as Rheumatoid arthritis or infections.

In other words, refined processed sugar creates the inflammatory occurrence even more rapidly.

Refined or processed sugar is not only served in many aliments we eat but it is served in excess. Excess sugar contributes to weight gain and excess body fat.

---

[6] https://www.uchicagomedicine.org/forefront/gastrointestinal-articles/2020/september/what-foods-cause-or-reduce-inflammation.

Excess body fat is known to participate in inflammation which ultimately leads to insulin resistance. In fact, according to the NIH, insulin resistance induced by inflammation is rising proportionally to the obesity pandemic.[7] Side Note:[8]

Refined Carbohydrates: Firstly, they are void of most nutrients thanks to the refining process, (we talked about processed foods above). They also have all kinds of additives such as trans fats, and refined sugars which lead to inflammation thanks to the disruption to our gut bacteria as just explained.

Dairy Products: There is conflicting information about this. This is where I feel dairy sensitivity may come into play but also in moderation. Moreover, the kinds of products on the shelves are at times questionable because dairy products are often pasteurized. Pasteurization destroys enzymes, diminishes vitamin content, and denatures fragile milk proteins. Also, dairy products are high in saturated fats. Saturated fats are known to participate in inflammation by directly stimulating the inflammation of our adipose (fat) tissue.

I asked myself, what type of dairy and how much of it was drank in biblical times? Well, they had curds of cows and milk of the flock - Deuteronomy 32:13-14. They had milk as a source of hydration Judge 4:19 - goat milk, and sheep cheese - 2 Samuel 17:29, Prov 27:27, etc… So they had many dairy foods when they had access!

However, dairy wasn't pasteurized and processed today as it was in biblical times or even back in our great grandfather's era. According to *Living History Farms*[9], pasteurization didn't start until

---

[7] https://www.ncbi.nlm.nih.gov/pmc/articles/PMC1483173/.

[8] I was comparing the label of Fanta Orange while in Togo, to US Fanta. The content of sugar per serving in Togo is 4.3g. The content of sugar in the US is 44g for the serving. My brother, made the same remark about pop while in Morocco.

[9] A museum about farming located in Urbandal, Iowa.

1862. The process of pasteurization makes it easier to digest dairy products. Dairy consumption was probably moderate in the past due to the difficulty in digesting it, which naturally limited intake.

Beyond the debate of dairy pasteurization and other processes, I am talking about the quantity we intake in today's society and its effect on our body in terms of inflammation. Again, **MODERATION**. So we easily introduce inflammation to our body by way of the things we eat, and in some cases inappropriate quantity of the things we eat

Alcohol: Sugar and Purine. We know how sugar participates in inflammation. The purine, however, participates in a different type of joint inflammation: Gout. Those who are not able to eliminate purine well, often deal with gout attacks.

Basically, by eating certain foods in excess or even exposing our bodies to certain foods we put our body in a state of inflammation. Never mind the issues already going on with our environment, and the process of oxidative stress that is behind any disease (for example LDL in itself is not harmless, however when it goes through the oxidative stress it creates those plaques that clog our arteries). A body in a state of inflammation is a free-for-all ground for oxidative stress. Inflammation is behind many diseases that plague our existence, and I can go on and on. Indeed inflammation is a curse as it is a basis for different types if not all diseases.

So I ask you again are you *"cursing"* yourself? As you can note, moderation is critical. **"Don't be greedy, for a greedy person is an idolater and worshipping the things of this world." Ephesians 5:5 NLT**. However, even if you can eat in moderation, is everything you eat beneficial to you and your health?

Interesting fact: Only mankind drinks animal milk past infancy, and only mankind drinks the milk of other species.

APPLICATION:

- Ask the Lord to reveal to you the foods you should eliminate or minimize from your diet. You also want to ask for the strength and ability to follow HIS recommendations. If you notice a pattern of this behavior in your family, especially down the generations; you want to address that (refer to a God-inspired deliverance book and/or Godly deliverance minister). Start from what you know but ask Him. He knows what your genetic predisposition is.

- Eliminate or minimize the foods that cause inflammation (start from what you know, and the conviction the Lord puts in your heart).

- The Bible reminds us in 2 Corinthians 10:4-7 the desire will come, but you want to "cast down any thoughts or imaginations that exalt itself against the knowledge of God and bring it into captivity to the obedience of Christ."- paraphrased. At some point, the devil just flees with those temptations, as you will not give in.

OBESITY AND INFAMMATION: When you are obese your body is in a continuous state of inflammation. Obesity is called metabolic inflammation.[10]

This is because excess fat promotes the increase of inflammatory factors. This leads to the condition called metabolic syndrome; the cluster of risk factors that put you at risk for cardiovascular diseases such as hypertension, high cholesterol, insulin resistance, prediabetes, diabetes (before being diabetic, you were prediabetic, before being found prediabetic, you were

---

[10] https://www.ncbi.nlm.nih.gov/pmc/articles/PMC8967417/.

insulin resistant). The need to adopt a lifestyle that promotes health is a survival necessity for mankind. The fact that available choices of nutrition promote the worst choices for you is simply wicked. God would not put in place a system that is destructive to His creation that He loves so much.

5

Skipping Menses by Artificial Means (contraceptives)

Did you know that oral contraceptives, especially those higher in estrogen can be a secondary cause of hypertension?

If you must be on contraceptives, my recommendation is to be on one that still allows the natural cycle. Why is that? Because every time we make unnatural choices with our body there are always outcomes or consequences that follow one way or another. Our body was designed a certain way and for a specific reason. Every time we go against God's natural order, we should not be surprised when we are dealing with negative consequences. Keep in mind though that with contraceptives you are still introducing hormones to your body.

The Creator is perfect, His work is perfect. I am always tickled by mankind's obsession with changing God's natural course of things (because there is also an evil course). If God created a certain process of operation for our body (which is fearfully and wonderfully made by the way) do you think He did not know what He was doing? Oh, how mankind loves to think of himself as wise in his own eyes!

Some ladies must undergo D&C (dilation and curettage) for the simple fact that their uterine lining does not shed as it is supposed to during their menses. Some others would take hormones to prevent the whole shedding occurrence; interesting, right? Now, one must stop such treatment if they decide they want to have children. But are you confident that the months off of taking birth control (injection, oral, patch, etc.....) before conception truly allowed those uterine walls to shed off many more months or years of thickening when it hasn't been shedding off? The shedding of the uterine wall (which is the menses we see) is a form of cleansing of the uterus. Therefore, preventing that process is similar to not cleaning your house for Lord knows how many months, and then doing one regular cleaning as opposed to a deep clean.

Normally, birth control prevents the uterine from thickening, that's one of the ways you do not get pregnant, that's the general understanding. However, note that the actual reality is that the uterine wall doesn't become as thick to favor an egg implantation. There is still some thickening occurring while on birth control. Also note that endometrium hyperplasia (overgrowth of the endometrium i.e. uterine wall) is caused by too much estrogen and not enough progesterone.

According to the ***Cleveland Clinic,*** some complications of amenorrhea (absence of menses) are difficulty getting pregnant, cardiovascular disease, and osteoporosis.[11]

---

[11] https://my.clevelandclinic.org/health/diseases/3924-amenorrhea.

Let me also say that the birth control you take to skip menses typically suppresses hormones (LH and FSH). This not only inhibits ovulation but also alters cervical mucus and endometrium.

The role of LH is to promote the differentiation of endometrial fibroblast (immature endometrial cells) into fully differentiated cells (mature cells) which are needed for implantation. Note that most cancerous cells are poorly differentiated cells. So, suppressing LH prevents the full differentiation of your cells every month. Now, you are repeating that over time while you are on birth control.

Let's take it from a Spiritual perspective.

1 Samuel 6:4 NKJV – "Then they said, What is the trespass offering which we shall return to Him? "They answered, "Five golden rats according to the number of the Lords of the Philistines. For the same plague was on all of you and your lords." This was in the context of the Philistines taking the Ark of the Lord and the plague that ensued (tumors and rats). They called on their magicians to figure out how to return the Ark and get rid of the curse. Another translation for the word tumor is emrod in the KJV which denotes "swell" or "mound." In other words, a growth with an inflammatory behavior. Note: the word *"inflammatory"* is again highlighted. From a medical perspective, we consider tumors to be cysts, fibroids, hemorrhoids (swollen and inflamed anal and rectal veins) as well as cancerous growth.

Deuteronomy 28:27[(a)] NLT - "The Lord will afflict you with the boils of Egypt and with tumors, scurvy, and the itch, from which you cannot be cured."

KJV – "The Lord will smite thee with the botch of Egypt, and with the emerods, and with the scab, and with the itch, whereof thou canst not be healed."

1 Samuel 5:6 NIV – "The Lord's hand was heavy on the people of Ashdod and its vicinity; he brought devastation on them and afflicted them with tumors."

NLT – "Then the Lord's heavy hand struck the people of Ashdod and the nearby villages with a plague of tumors."

1 Samuel 5:9 NIV – "But after they had moved it, the Lord's hand was against that city, throwing it into a great panic. He afflicted the men of the city, both young and old, with an outbreak of tumors."

1 Samuel 5:12 NIV – "Those who did not die were afflicted with tumors, and the outcry of the city went up to heaven."

NLT – "Those who didn't die were afflicted with tumors, and the cry from the town rose to heaven."

You get it, tumors are a curse, it is an affliction, it doesn't have to be cancer.

Adopting a behavior that promotes a process that participates in the occurrence of tumors (poor cell differentiation) is just as giving the enemy a free ride. It also occurred to me that a mother herself may not deal with the consequences in her lifetime, but this thing can manifest later down the road by the principle of Epigenetics. Yes, this is a generational cursing behavior.

On a side note, I realize the level of pride, arrogance, defiance, and blatant self-idolization when indulging in behaviors that *"create"* a curse. Many also do this out of ignorance: *"Lord although I am not doing what they did in the Old Testament to bring the curse of all sorts of tumors on them, what I am going to do is take medications to increase my likelihood of creating those tumors. I will then blame You or ask You why this is happening to me or my bloodline?"*

Note, I realize that some individual's lifestyles may require them to skip menses (pro athletes, especially swimmers), however, this shouldn't be an ongoing matter from my perspective, frankly, this is a discussion you should have with God. Hence the importance of an intimate relationship with Him so you will know what He is telling you.

I asked the Lord to delay my menses for a long trip I was taking, and He answered. The minute I arrived; my menses started.

You may exclaim, *"I do not take anything to have an irregular cycle."* I could relate until I received an understanding that it should not be that way and what I had to do about it.

To answer you, I would like to ask you why is your cycle irregular? What is your lifestyle like? Stress level? Stress management. One of the many reasons for irregular menses besides actual medical conditions such as pituitary disorders, is often lifestyle. There may also be a genetic component regardless as a believer, this is something to address both in the natural and in prayer. For instance, those dealing with PCOS [12] are often dealing with insulin resistance (it is believed by science to be greatly involved in this whole PCOS issue). Interestingly enough, a mechanism behind insulin resistance is inflammation from excess fat.[13]

If you are curious about how I was able to regulate my cycles, I changed what, how, and why I ate. I started exercising, and weight loss occurred naturally. I will also say that it has been a road of inner healing, and deliverance, as well as confronting

---

[12] Polycystic Ovarian Syndrome (PCOS)

[13] https://www.ncbi.nlm.nih.gov/pmc/articles/PMC1483173/#:~:text=Increasing%20adiposity%20activates%20inflammatory%20responses,these%20cause%20local%20insulin%20resistance.

and addressing faulty foundations

As previously noted, when you are obese your body is in a continuous state of inflammation. If you have a lifestyle that promotes inflammation this would be something to address.

The Role of STRESS

I cannot *stress* this enough: the state of your mental health influences your hormonal behavior.

When I mention lifestyle, I mean all aspects of your life including the sexual aspect. Promiscuity and multiple partners only introduce all kinds of spirits in you. Do I need to elaborate on this? Let me stick to the purpose of this book.

SIDE NOTE. As a teenager, it dawned on me that natural birthing occurs through the vagina, the same organ necessary for sex. Now the creation of sex was for a man and woman to be one, hence the introduction of your partner's spirits to you when you sleep with them; you become one spiritually.

That contact occurs in the vagina canal. Ladies, your children are supposed to pass through that canal too. Keep it clean and without spiritual contaminants. Those spiritual contaminants are patiently waiting for that child to be conceived. They have legal grounds through fornication or promiscuity. Your future child is pretty much an innocent victim. Not only that, they can easily travel to your other organs.

6

Autoimmune Conditions

According to **The National Institute of Health** *"A healthy immune system defends the body against disease and infection (and yes, the immune response often involves inflammation to rid of the foreign or bad/defective elements)."* But then again if the immune system malfunctions, it mistakenly attacks healthy cells, tissues, and organs. Called *"autoimmune diseases,"* these attacks can affect any part of the body, weakening bodily function and even becoming life-threatening. It goes on to say that there are over 80 autoimmune conditions that science has identified so far.[14]

Autoimmune conditions such as RA, psoriasis, and type I diabetes (pancreatic cell destruction) are a matter of your body's immune system attacking the very host of said immune system: self-destruction. Although an autoimmune condition may not necessarily be lethal when left untreated (i.e. vitiligo), the very

---

14 The National Institute of Health. https://www.niehs.nih.gov/health/topics/conditions/autoimmune/index.cfm.

concept of the body attacking itself calls for some questions with several question marks. Not only does it point to some sort of error in the system, but also to a system's confusion.

Since the role of the immune system is to protect the body from invading hosts, an autoimmune situation would denote that the body is essentially protecting itself from itself by attacking itself. Could there be something in the organ with the autoimmune condition that is triggering the immune response against it; or identifying that organ as foreign? In which case the immune response is legitimate and the question would be how is that organ *"foreign"* to the body? Or did something trigger the immune system to confuse its host as being a pathogen or foreign?

I believe that autoimmune conditions are also a way of telling us that in the spiritual realm, there may be a presence or contention against your very being or existence. Although an autoimmune reaction is an error per science definition; **God** doesn't make errors. Moreover, if anything that takes place in the natural has already taken place in the spirit, there has been an *"anti-you"* occurrence in the spirit. The question is how did that occurrence take place? Remember I mentioned that the choices we make may not show forth consequences in our lifetime, but later in our bloodline. Note that this would then apply to all aspects of life, but this book is about the nutritional aspect. Although I trust that it will give you a specific revelation for other aspects of your life.

I also believe that there may be a component of autoimmunity when the actual organ is not acting the way it is supposed to which will make the immune system consider it foreign since it is not acting as supposed to.

Let's make sense of autoimmunity scripturally.

Self-Destruction: 2 Chronicles 20: 22-24 NLT - "At the very moment they began to sing and give praise, the LORD caused the armies of Ammon, Moab, and Mount Seir to start fighting among themselves. The armies of Moab and Ammon turned against their allies from Mount Seir and killed every one of them. After they had destroyed the army of Seir, they began attacking each other. So when the army of Judah arrived at the lookout point in the wilderness, all they saw were dead bodies lying on the ground as far as they could see. Not a single one of the enemy had escaped."

Confusion: 1 Corinthians 14:13 NKJV – "For God is not *the author* of confusion but of peace, as in all the churches of the saints."

Deuteronomy 7:23 NLT - "But the LORD your God will hand them over to you. He will throw them into complete confusion until they are destroyed."

Confusion is for the enemy. Meaning if you are an enemy of God confusion is part of your portion. Is there something about your life or in your existence that makes you an enemy of God therefore translating confusion into the very biological processes of your body as an autoimmune condition?

Am I saying you are an enemy of God? Not necessarily; however, there are things in your life, lifestyle, and nutritional pattern that give the devil all sorts of arguments to accuse you in the throne room and to have legal grounds to carry out the curses that come with whatever the acts of disobedience, sin, iniquity, and even ignorance which have already been put in place. There may be something that makes you an abomination to God.

When you read the scriptures, confusion is served to those against God, His Will, and His children. Confusion is directed towards the enemy of God: James 4:4.[15]

There is something that is an adversary to your body to act toward itself as its own enemy. This is something that can only occur by confusion. Confusion is for the enemies of God and His children in other words there is a basis that is not of God. Now let me say this:

Could the condition be due to some issue during the formation of the baby in the womb, or his/her development in the womb?

Could it be due to the quality of sperm and egg that formed that child?

I do not negate the fact that whatever it is could have also been projected by way of a curse with a legal ground through trauma, sin, or iniquity. However, as far as this book is concerned, we are looking at nutritional lifestyles and auto-immune diseases.

Hosea 4:6 KJV - "My people are destroyed for lack of knowledge: because thou hast rejected knowledge, I will also reject thee, that thou shalt be no priest to me: seeing thou hast forgotten the law of thy God, I will also forget thy children." Forgetting, and ignoring the need to acquire Godly knowledge goes with rejecting knowledge.

"Reject" in Hebrew is Ma'as which means to despise, refuse.

According to the NIH, "Nutrition and immunity are closely related, and the immune system is composed of the most

---

15 James 4:4 NIV - You adulterous people,[a] don't you know that friendship with the world means enmity against God? Therefore, anyone who chooses to be a friend of the world becomes an enemy of God.

highly energy-consuming cells in the body[16]. Much of the immune system is located within the GI tract… Moreover, the incidence of immune-mediated diseases is elevated in Westernized countries, where *"transition nutrition"* prevails, owing to the shift from traditional dietary patterns towards Westernized patterns."

Transition Nutrition: The alterations in dietary patterns, levels of physical activity, and factors contributing to diseases that occur alongside shifts in economic development, lifestyle, urbanization, and demographic trends.

Science recognizes a link between diet and autoimmune disease, but it hasn't fully explained it, however. Through diet, one can challenge or aid the proper functioning of one's immune system. When you reflect on the chapters above, also through diet, one could simply be introducing a curse into their lives or even bloodline.

Through diet, you can turn your body into its enemy. Remember that the devil only comes to steal, kill, and destroy. So with the wrong eating lifestyle, you are helping the devil be successful in his mission, he is probably giving you all the bad choices and pieces of advice anyway; he is the worst advisor.

The plan of **God** is not for us to live miserable sick, frail, etc. The Bible references those who died *"strong"* and not frail. This pattern we see around us today is not the plan of our **Heavenly Father.**

---

[16] This is the reason why you are more likely to get sick if you have been tired for a while.

One may say, *"Well my child has done nothing to deal with autoimmune conditions."* This is where generation or bloodline matters are at hand. Reflecting on the previous chapters can help you identify because of this issue.

Sometimes, it is through exposure to certain toxins or medications that one finds oneself suddenly coming up with new symptoms and is diagnosed with an autoimmune disease.

The relationship between our food choices and our gut health was mentioned earlier in this chapter. A lot of our autoimmune system relies on our gut health. There are many vitamins such as the B vitamin involved in immune functions. Consider the consequences of a generational deficit of the B vitamins and how it would affect immune functions.

APPLICATION:

Repent for eating choices you know are not right. Repent for the generations before you; and change your ways. Be determined to change your ways, and make the decision not to be an easy victim of the enemy.

Cannibalism

If you are aware that cannibalism was practiced in your bloodline; Repent, Renounce, and Replace: Genesis 9:3-6, Leviticus 26:29, Ezekiel 5: 10, and Jeremiah 19:9. As referenced in these scriptures, God forbade cannibalism. It was a terrible judgment for wickedness and disobedience towards God. If you know cannibalism was practiced in your bloodline, you need to address it. Let the Lord tell you how.

7

Epigenetics

Epigenetics: [17] *"The study of heritable changes in gene function that do not involve changes in* DNA *sequence."* Note that the DNA sequence does not change but the gene function does. For example, the fat-burning gene (UCP1) may learn to burn less fat, etc… or the insulin-regulating gene (INS gene) may be less active than it needs to be. The key takeaway here is that the change in gene function is passed down to generation. The gene itself may not change, but its job or the accuracy and efficiency of its job may change.

Adoption Studies: Twin studies and twin-adoption studies have supported the role of genetics in obesity. This is where the concept of epigenetics becomes crucial. When you think about it before the existence of today's modern transportation, mankind was very active and physically fit thanks to his daily life. Over time, obesity started taking place as we decided to make it easier and faster in all aspects of our lives along with the introduction of particular foods and our eating habits. As we adjust to our

[17] Epigenetics: definition per Merriam Webster Dictionary.

environment, so do our genes, and it is passed down to our children generations beyond.

A very popular study by *Dr. Claude Bouchard* of Canada showed that when a sample of individuals were overfed the same amount of calories, they all gained different amounts of weight: some subjects only gained 4 kgs while others gained 13 kgs. In other words, everybody gains weight differently. The study also noted that the weight gain was similar for identical twins as opposed to fraternal twins. This is where having intimacy with the Lord and seeking His guidance in our eating habits becomes critical.

Here is a motivation for wanting to adopt a lifestyle that aligns with the health of your body, mind, and soul as intended by God: **It gets passed down.**

In other words, the concept of generational curse is transcribed in our bloodline. You may say well, is obesity a curse? I invite you to read Judges 3:17, Deuteronomy 32:15, Jeremiah 5:28, Psalm 73.7, 1 Samuel 2: 29. Note that the individuals that were referred to as fat were not pleasing to the Almighty in their behaviors and drew judgment and curses on themselves. This is because of the way they got fat!

So, today, by idolizing food, technology, and modernization, we become fat.

Let me explain something, when you choose to drive to a place half a mile from your location as opposed to walking there (unless conditions do not permit) you are idolizing your modern transportation over walking or biking which would be the God way. Why? Because He designed our bodies to MOVE and be active. Adam had to tend to the garden after being created. That was laborious work if you ask me. What motivates our choice to drive very short distances, aside from specific limitations? Laziness and an excessive reliance on the comfort of our cars come to mind. We have become overly dependent on them. It might also be that the weariness from the burdens of this world leads to seeking solace in the ease of driving, the only place where you can catch a break.

There is an evil spiritual assignment that influences those who find themselves overindulging in food, ignoring the need to stay a minimum active, and so on. Again, this doesn't apply to fatness from medical conditions such as endocrine issues. However, I would invite you to look at the Inflammatory chapter (4) as far as those very conditions that put you in that undesirable position.

I will also remark that I do not agree with the definition of fat always correlating with a BMI. The weight and BMI of bodybuilders challenge that theory. When you are carrying an excess weight of fat you know it. I will also point out that fat does play an important role in our body (some hormonal balance for example) some fat is healthy. I am referring to excessive fat as being the issue.

Here is what I am trying to tell you: be motivated to teach your genes their proper function by how you treat your body despite the mass initiation of self-destruction going on. (1 Corinthians 6:19).

8

The Subtly Promoted Sedentary Lifestyle

As mentioned in the previous chapter, society is designed to make things easier and faster. Why? To give you time. You typically use that time for what? To give it back to whatever society is demanding, such as perhaps a time-abusive job, being idle, etc... We do not even use the extra time for God because that time is taken by all the demands of this modern society.

I was born and raised in West Africa. Every time I go home and interact with other professionals, I am flabbergasted by the amount of time available for other meaningful activities, such as family, etc… unless they choose to work in so many places. In the US it seems there is never enough time for anything. So for the sake of time, we have means of transportation that allow us to reach distant destinations much faster. We have eliminated daily physical activities that we would have otherwise gotten years ago by walking to catch the bus. Unless one is mindful of investing time in physical activities (gym, fitness classes, walking, swimming, etc…), one is otherwise sedentary.

Isn't it interesting that the very society that is telling you to be healthy is designed in such a way to also promote the lack of activity? One thing that amazes me when I read the Bible is the physical capability of those whose stories are told. The amount of walking, and the distances they traveled! Thank God we can travel distances they traveled in months within hours. But then, what do we use the extra time for?

What happens when you're physically active? According to Mayo Clinic, it helps control weight, combats health conditions and diseases, improves mood, boosts energy, improves sleep, and puts a spark in your sexual life (for married folks). According to the NIH, the mechanism at the basis of those benefits *"not only drives healthy adaptations but also antagonizes the inflammation and metabolic consequences of atrophy and aging. Exercise increases the expression of key adaptive genes and promotes the secretion of molecules that signal adaptive responses in various tissues and slows age-related decline."* [18]

Basically, by not exercising, we shouldn't complain we are aging faster, our body is struggling to adapt to some changes, or we are dealing with inflammation. So, do you see how the lack of activity or promotion of a sedentary lifestyle only makes the enemy camp happier as far as your existence goes? It is like handing him the knife he will use to execute you: slowly and miserably.

---

[18]https://www.ncbi.nlm.nih.gov/pmc/articles/PMC9462916/#:~:text=These%20mechanisms%20not%20only%20drive,and%20slows%20age%2Drelated%20decline .

According to the CDC *"Being physically active can improve your brain health, reduce stress, strengthen bones and muscles, and improve your ability to do everyday activities. Adults who sit less and do any amount of moderate-to-vigorous physical activity gain some health benefits.* ***Only a few lifestyle choices have as large an impact on your health as physical activity."***[19]

[19] https://www.cdc.gov/physicalactivity/basics/pa-health/index.htm#:~:text=Being%20physically%20active%20can%20improve,activity%20gain%20some%20health%20benefits. https://newsnetwork.mayoclinic.org/discussion/7-benefits-of-regular-physical-activity/.

9

A Quick Note On Mental Health: Depression and Anxiety

I am specifically talking about depression and anxiety not only because of their commonality in the Bible believer's population but also because the other conditions are more specific and specialized. The quality of nutrition is directly correlated to mood. When you eat junk food, it is easy for depression to follow.[20] Unfortunately, depression and anxiety walk hand in hand. When you are not despondent, you are overly afraid and worried or both! I explained earlier how a poor nutritional lifestyle is grounds for you cursing yourself, opening doors for demons and evil spirits to operate in your life legally. Understand that it applies also to depression and anxiety.

According to the American Nutrition Society, a healthy diet provides more vitamins and minerals, healthy fats, and fiber from fruits, vegetables, whole grains, nuts, and seeds, which can reduce inflammation and alter neurotransmitters to reduce

---

[20] *Many of the chemicals in artificial ingredients affect your mood negatively.*

symptoms of depression. On a spiritual level, the very food God made available to us for nutrition helps guard us against evil invaders when eaten the right way and in the right amount. Genesis 1:30.

10

Fasting

The power of fasting is undeniable. There are several books dedicated to this topic. Throughout the scriptures, we saw the children of Israel and even Jesus engage in fasts. The results that stem from those fasts showed how the fasts in question not only strengthened, aligned, and empowered the one fasting to face and dominate the challenges, opposition, or trial they were facing but most importantly gave them victory over their enemies. Isaiah 58 is very clear about why and how we should fast. Nowhere does it mention that we fast to influence God's decision or to get God to do something for us. According to Isaiah 58 fasting truly realigns us with God and propels us in a position where we can step into the will and purpose of God.

I have struggled with excess weight since I could walk as my Mom would say. I grew up sick. I was always sick. When I sat in my Primary Care Provider's (PCP) office and received the news that I had to go on blood pressure medications because my blood pressure was out of control, I told myself "There was no way."

High blood pressure ran aggressively in my bloodline and I was not going to start on that path.

I was put on metformin for diabetes. Due to my being overweight (obese), since I was a little girl, there have been several attempts at weight loss. There were several defeating, depressing attempts to help me to lose weight. Whenever I would lose some weight; it was always short-lived.

After I visited with my PCP, I went home and told God *"This life of sickness and medications is not what you desire for your children. I do not understand why things are how they are but I need your help."* So, I went on a fast asking God to help me to become what He intended me to be when he designed and created me. After all, I knew His way was the right way and it had nothing to do with emotional or stress eating, constant malaise, or constant sickness. This is how my successful weight loss journey started. I went to an endocrinologist to investigate the potential hormonal causes behind my obesity.

The provider ran basic tests (which I had done several times before and it always came back normal); he decided to put me on weight loss medications. I decided to comply and began taking the medication, but it only lasted for one month due to how it made me feel.

After my body rejected the medication, I went on the Fast God instructed me to do. At the end of the fast, my relationship with food changed. Do not misunderstand me, I am a foodie, I love good food, and I like to try all sorts of foods from different cultures. However, I realized that I was now in control of my eating, as opposed to the food having control over me.

I also noticed that I was more aware of my emotional state and challenged it quickly with prayer when thoughts or negative feelings tried to influence my eating. For example, I would have a plate in front of me and would spontaneously understand the portions on my plate and how I should change them. I would put things on my plate and the **Holy Spirit** would instruct me to look those things up. Sometimes, **He** would say *"Don't eat that"* or "*That is too much."* The **Holy Spirit** was and remains my personal weight loss coach! **He** definitively gave me instructions on eating.

This is how I started gaining serious interest in looking up foods, or aliments and how they may help or challenge me. I did try the weight loss medications as mentioned for a brief moment but I hated the side effects so much I only tried it for a few weeks (which I never admitted to the endocrinologist).

I used to hate to exercise, but I joined a gym because I knew I also needed to exercise. A personal trainer approached me at the gym and offered four free workout sessions. Due to my prior experiences with personal trainers, I was very defensive and almost missed a blessing; but things were so different with *"Coach."* This turned out to be an individual whom I believe has a true calling on his life to help individuals on their health journey.

It has been years since training with "Coach" and now exercising is of high importance to me. If I don't exercise at least 4 days a week, my focus, healthy eating, and sleep suffer significantly and depression is like a snare crouching at my door to attack my body and mind. **Genesis 4-7 NIV.**

According to science, fasting allows our body to cleanse but also reset and regenerate. It helps *"recalibrate"* our body. Abstaining from food (how did intermittent fasting become so popular?) creates that effect. Isn't it interesting that as far as a scriptural fast, this helps you realign with **God**? Have you noticed how easily you hear from the **Lord** during a fast? (Of course, I am talking about abstaining from food or some types of food fast). Some get inspiration and revelations during the fast. So what happens in the spirit during a fast is so powerful that it tangibly translates into the physical for even science to measure and validate it. From that validation, fasting is to the point where it is now promoted far from its original biblical purpose.

11

CONCLUSION

I have this picture of a mass initiation through the foods that are being produced and fed to us, especially in the US and the Western World. This has also been gaining ground in Africa. I dare not talk about the other parts of the world since I haven't been there yet, but I remain highly suspicious that it is occurring everywhere. The level of processing of the food and the pathetic standard behind it in the USA as opposed to other developed countries is just embarrassing. I still appreciate the fact that I am mostly eating organic food when I go home, although the agenda to advance GMOs is gaining ground on the continent.

3 John 1:2 KJV "Beloved, I pray that you may prosper in all things and be in health just as your soul prospers." What is the state of your soul?

I think that it is critical to go to the root of anything you know is not from God and destroy it there. Ask yourself why do I behave in a way that treats the temple of God anyhow? When you go to the Church Building, you do not go around throwing trash all over the place and so on. You wouldn't do that to a structure made of lifeless materials yet, you would do it to yourself who is fearfully and wonderfully made in **His Image.** You are **His** child in whom **He** breathed the breath of life for you to walk this earth. Beyond that, you should also ask **Him** to reveal to you the causes of why you are destroying your body, especially when you find yourself struggling with self-control. Many will find they need deliverance, inner healing, perhaps even counseling (really tied to inner healing), and growth in the **Lord.** Many of you may find their intimacy with the **Lord** is not where it should have been by now or is perhaps nonexistent. Many of you may find they have been living in religion as opposed to in a relationship with the **Lord.**

This book is mostly for those who are trying to make sense of how the spiritual plays into nutrition, and how it ultimately plays a part in our destiny on earth. We cannot declare and proclaim that we will fulfill the number of our days if we cook every single recipe for heart attacks, hypertension, strokes, and diabetes. We cannot proclaim that **Jesus** bore our sicknesses while chasing down the sicknesses, inviting them into our bodies, and ensuring they are comfortable (really, the spirits of infirmity and death).

I pray this book stirs you enough to decide to become a health-conscious Believer.

1 Corinthians 10:23 NKJV:

"All things are lawful for me, but not all things are helpful, all things are lawful for me but not all things edify."

ABOUT THE AUTHOR

Rachel's roots in Togo, West Africa, imbue her journey with a rich cultural backdrop and a deep appreciation for health and wellness. Rachel's journey is a testament to the transformative power of personal experience and passion in shaping one's career path. Despite initially intending to pursue medicine, her exposure to the hospital environment in the US led her to discover a profound love for nursing. This shift was not only influenced by her fascination with healthcare but also by practical considerations such as the cost of medical school.

Starting with an associate degree in nursing, Rachel's dedication and commitment to her profession propelled her to further her education, eventually earning a Bachelor of Science in Nursing (BSN) and then a Master of Science in Nursing (MSN). Her journey culminated in becoming a Nurse Practitioner in 2017, a role that allowed her to expand her scope of practice and delve deeper into disease prevention and health promotion.

Rachel's passion for holistic health and wellness is evident in her company, Shalem Lifestyle, where she offers Health Coaching services. Through her own health experiences and spiritual journey, Rachel discovered the profound impact of nutrition beyond its surface value. This realization, coupled with her faith, guided her toward a deeper understanding of the interconnectedness between physical, mental, and spiritual well-being.

Many years ago, on a bright and sunny day, Rachel found herself longing for a specific type of potato chip. Despite being committed to a healthier lifestyle, the craving was strong and she decided to indulge. As she approached a gas station to buy them, Rachel felt a divine nudge questioning whether this desire was truly from Him. Fast forward to today, Rachel is now a published author.

When God first suggested to Rachel that she would write a book, she remembers laughing and saying, *"I had never been fond of writing."* Yet, she decided to challenge Him; if He wanted her to write about this topic, He would need to provide the structure. Remarkably, Rachel dreamt about all the chapters soon after.

www.ingramcontent.com/pod-product-compliance
Lightning Source LLC
LaVergne TN
LVHW010545100826
845148LV00013B/2608

* 9 7 9 8 2 1 8 4 2 5 2 7 2 *